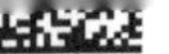

HERBAL REMEDIES FOR ERECTILE DYSFUNCTION

Revitalize Your Body's Machinery With Herbal Solutions For Optimal Health, Holistic Wellness And Guide To Rejuvenate Your Vital Systems Naturally

DR. CARDEN KYRIE

DISCLAIMER

The only goal of this book is informational. Every effort has been taken by the author and publisher to ensure that the information provided is accurate. But the material in this book is given "as is," without any express or implied representation, warranty, or condition as to its accuracy, completeness, or suitability for any particular purpose.

Any loss, damage, or injury resulting from using the information in this book, or from any action or decision made as a result of such use, will not be covered by the author's or publisher's liability. It is recommended that readers seek the assistance of a certified specialist for guidance specific to their situation.

The opinions and viewpoints conveyed in this book belong to the author and may not necessarily represent the official stance or policies of any specified organizations or people. Any likeness to real-life occurrences, places, or people—living or deceased—is wholly coincidental.

No specific product, service, or therapy discussed in this book is endorsed by the author or publisher. Any reference to goods or services is made only for informative reasons and is not intended as a recommendation or endorsement.

Before making any judgments or acting on any information, readers are urged to independently confirm it all. Any unfavorable effects or repercussions arising from the usage of the material included in this book are disclaimed by the author and publisher.

By using this book, you consent to absolving the publisher and author of any and all claims, obligations, or losses resulting from your use of the material in it.

I appreciate your cooperation and understanding.

TABLE OF CONTENTS

CHAPTER ONE 8

INTRODUCTION TO ERECTILE DYSFUNCTION.................................8

AN OVERVIEW OF PROBLEMS WITH ERECTION 8

THE VALUE OF LOOKING FOR NATURAL SOLUTIONS 9

CHAPTER TWO 12

KNOWLEDGE OF ERECTILE DYSFUNCTION 12

MEANING AND REASONS 12

PHYSICAL ELEMENTS 12

PSYCHOLOGICAL ELEMENTS..13

TYPICAL RISK ELEMENTS 14

THE IMPACT OF ERECTILE DYSFUNCTION ON PARTNERSHIPS 15

CHAPTER THREE 16

OVERVIEW OF HERBAL REMEDIES 16

BENEFITS OF USING HERBAL TREATMENTS 16

HERBS HAVE BEEN USED HISTORICALLY FOR SEXUAL HEALTH 17

REGULATION AND SAFETY OF HERBAL SUPPLEMENTS 17

CHAPTER FOUR 20

ESSENTIAL HERBS FOR IMPOTENCE 20

GINSENG PANAX 20

ADMINISTRATION & DOSAGE 20

GOAT HORN (EPIMEDIUM) WEED.....................................21

ADVANTAGES OF ERECTILE DYSFUNCTION 22

CHAPTER FIVE...24

THOUGHTS AND ADVERSE REACTIONS.................................24

INCREASING BLOOD FLOW..24

POSSIBLE RELATIONSHIPS 24

TERRESTRIS TRIBULUS 25

PROPERTIES THAT BOOST TESTOSTERONE 26

USAGE INSTRUCTIONS 26

CHAPTER SIX...28

RECIPES AND FORMULAS FOR HERBS 28

HERBAL TEAS FOR HEALTHY ERECTILE FUNCTION 28

EXTRACTS AND TINCTURES 29

BLENDS & SMOOTHIES USING HERBS 29

FORMULATING A CUSTOMIZED HERBAL REGIMEN 30

CHAPTER SEVEN 32

DIETARY GUIDELINES AND LIFESTYLE FACTORS 32

DIET'S IMPACT ON ERECTILE FUNCTION 32

FOODS THAT HELP WITH IMPOTENCE 32

FOODS TO STEER CLEAR OF...33

PHYSICAL ACTIVITY AND EXERCISE...34

TECHNIQUES FOR STRESS MANAGEMENT 34

CHAPTER EIGHT...36

COMBINING CONVENTIONAL AND CONTEMPORARY METHODS 36

BLENDING TRADITIONAL MEDICAL PROCEDURES WITH HERBAL
REMEDIES..36

SPEAKING WITH MEDICAL EXPERTS..37

TRACKING DEVELOPMENT AND MODIFYING APPROACHES 38

CHAPTER NINE 40

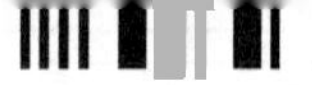

CASE STUDIES AND TRIUMPHANT NARRATIVES 40

ACTUAL HERBAL MEDICINE EXPERIENCES 40

ACQUIRED KNOWLEDGE AND UNDERSTANDING 41

RESOLVING FREQUENTLY ASKED QUESTIONS.....................................42

DISPELLING MYTHS REGARDING HERBAL TREATMENTS...................43

CHAPTER ONE

INTRODUCTION TO ERECTILE DYSFUNCTION

AN OVERVIEW OF PROBLEMS WITH ERECTION

An enormous number of men globally suffer from erectile dysfunction (ED), a medical illness that is common regardless of age, ethnicity, or socioeconomic status. The inability to consistently get or sustain an erection strong enough for satisfying sexual performance is what defines it. Beyond the physical, ED influences mental and emotional health as well, frequently leading to unhappiness and strained relationships.

Navigating the challenges of erectile dysfunction requires an understanding of its diverse nature. Many different variables can lead to eating disorders (ED), including psychological issues like stress, anxiety, and depression as well as physiological issues like diabetes, hormone imbalances, and cardiovascular diseases. A sedentary lifestyle, heavy alcohol use, and smoking are some of the lifestyle choices that greatly increase the occurrence of ED. Because of these complex interactions, prevention, and therapy must be approached from all angles.

People are starting to realize how important it is to look for natural solutions in the fight against erectile dysfunction. This change is motivated by a desire to investigate comprehensive and long-lasting remedies that deal with the root causes as well as the symptoms. Natural remedies cover a wide range of treatments, from herbal supplements and alternative therapies to dietary adjustments and lifestyle adjustments. Adopting natural therapies helps allay worries about possible negative effects linked with pharmaceutical interventions and also fits in with the current trend toward wellness-oriented methods.

THE VALUE OF LOOKING FOR NATURAL SOLUTIONS

The importance of looking for natural cures comes from the fact that they might improve general health and well-being. Natural therapies, in contrast to some pharmacological interventions, frequently take a holistic approach, addressing all facets of a person's health. Adopting healthy lifestyle practices, such as consistent exercise and eating a well-balanced diet, not only enhances sexual function but also improves hormone balance, cardiovascular health, and mental health. An expanded comprehension of the interdependence of several aspects of health and their influence on sexual vitality is reflected in this integrative approach.

The allure of natural therapies also stems from their apparent safety and lack of side effects. People are gravitating toward natural options because they believe they are kinder to their bodies than pharmaceutical therapies, especially as awareness of the possible hazards linked with them rises. A more subtle approach to treating erectile dysfunction is provided by herbal supplements, conventional treatments, and lifestyle changes without exposing patients to the possible side effects of prescription medications.

The field of treating erectile dysfunction is changing, with a focus on natural therapies and a holistic knowledge of the problem. The complex interactions between physiological and psychological components emphasize the necessity of all-encompassing strategies that go beyond treating symptoms. Adopting natural therapies underscores the significance of taking into account the interconnected components of health in the goal of sexual vitality, in addition to being in line with a larger trend towards holistic well-being.

CHAPTER TWO

KNOWLEDGE OF ERECTILE DYSFUNCTION MEANING AND REASONS

The inability to consistently get or sustain an erection strong enough for sexual activity is known as erectile dysfunction (ED). Men of all ages can be affected by this ailment, though it gets more common as people age. Erectile dysfunction is caused by a variety of reasons, which can be broadly divided into physical and psychological factors.

PHYSICAL ELEMENTS

Physical factors include a variety of illnesses and lifestyle decisions that can affect nerve activity and blood flow, both of which are essential for a good erection. Obesity, diabetes, thyroid abnormalities, cardiovascular disease, and neurological illnesses are common physical causes. A sedentary lifestyle,

smoking, and excessive alcohol intake are some lifestyle choices that might hasten the onset of ED.

Acknowledging the significance of a robust circulatory system is necessary to comprehend the physiological elements associated with ED. Atherosclerosis, a disorder characterized by the hardening and constriction of the arteries, can obstruct blood flow to the penis, making it more difficult to obtain an erection. Erectile dysfunction can result from neurological conditions like multiple sclerosis that disrupt signals that are sent from the brain to the genital area.

PSYCHOLOGICAL ELEMENTS

Erectile dysfunction is mostly caused by psychological issues, which are frequently linked to physical causes. Psychological variables such as stress, worry, sadness, and relationship problems can either cause or worsen eating disorders (ED). The complex relationship between mental health and sexual function is highlighted by the fact that mental health disorders can impact the brain's capacity to send signals that initiate and sustain an erection.

Erectile dysfunction is influenced by psychological variables that stem from the intricate relationship between the brain and body. Stress and worry can cause the release of hormones like cortisol, which can hurt sexual function. These hormones can be related to the job, performance, or personal life. ED can also be exacerbated by depression, a widespread mood illness that impairs libido and general enthusiasm for sexual activity.

TYPICAL RISK ELEMENTS

An increased chance of developing erectile dysfunction is typically linked to several risk factors. One important determinant is age; as men age, the prevalence of ED increases. Other risk factors include not getting enough exercise daily, smoking, drinking too much alcohol, and being obese.

Diabetes and cardiovascular disorders are two chronic medical problems that increase the chance of having ED.

THE IMPACT OF ERECTILE DYSFUNCTION ON PARTNERSHIPS

Relationships can be significantly impacted by erectile dysfunction in ways that go beyond physical closeness. Both partners may experience severe emotional consequences, including feelings of annoyance, inadequacy, and a weakened sense of connection. To overcome the difficulties presented by ED, partners must be able to communicate openly to develop empathy and understanding. The emotional toll that erectile dysfunction takes on relationships can be effectively addressed by seeking expert assistance, such as couples therapy or counseling.

Realizing the complexity of erectile dysfunction's origins is essential to comprehending the condition.

CHAPTER THREE

OVERVIEW OF HERBAL REMEDIES

BENEFITS OF USING HERBAL TREATMENTS

The extensive use of herbal treatments can be attributed to their perceived benefits and holistic approach to health and well-being. Herbal treatments' natural source, which is typically plants, flowers, roots, or other botanical materials, is one of its main advantages. Herbal treatments, as opposed to synthetic drugs, are believed to function in tandem with the body to facilitate a gradual and well-rounded healing process. The fact that natural therapies frequently have fewer adverse effects than pharmaceutical options is something that many individuals find appealing.

Furthermore, compared to conventional drugs, herbal medicines are frequently more easily obtained and reasonably priced. Herbal knowledge has been passed down through the generations in a variety of cultures, enabling people to make use of the medicinal qualities of plants that are easily found in their surroundings. By making common health issues more accessible, communities can manage them on their own without depending entirely on contemporary medicine.

HERBS HAVE BEEN USED HISTORICALLY FOR SEXUAL HEALTH

Many ancient civilizations recognized the therapeutic effects of some plants in increasing reproductive health and vitality, and for ages, they used herbs to promote sexual health. Herbs have long been used in traditional Chinese medicine, Ayurveda, and other indigenous healing systems to treat problems related to sexual health. Herbs such as ginseng, maca root, and ashwagandha.

REGULATION AND SAFETY OF HERBAL SUPPLEMENTS

The growing popularity of herbal treatments has brought greater importance to the safety and regulation of these supplements. Although most people believe herbal medicines to be natural and safe, it's important to understand that not all plants are risk-free or without adverse effects. Inconsistencies in the effects of herbal products might arise from differences in quality and the absence of defined dosages. Regulatory agencies are essential in guaranteeing the security and caliber of herbal supplements. That being said, laws about herbal treatments might differ greatly between nations.

Herbal supplements could have difficulties with quality control and standardized testing in some areas where they are not as closely regulated as pharmaceutical pharmaceuticals. Therefore, before adding herbal items to their wellness regimens, consumers are advised to get them from reliable suppliers and seek medical advice. This cautious approach guarantees that people are aware of the advantages and disadvantages of using herbal treatments and helps reduce the possibility of problems with other medications.

The benefits of using herbal treatments are their natural source, ease of use, and supposedly low negative effects. Herbs have traditionally been used for sexual health, indicating a long-standing understanding of their potential advantages in enhancing reproductive health. To guarantee the caliber and effectiveness of these natural treatments, regulatory bodies must continuously monitor the safety and regulation of herbal supplements, which highlights the importance of educated consumer decision-making.

CHAPTER FOUR

ESSENTIAL HERBS FOR IMPOTENCE

GINSENG PANAX

The possible health advantages of Panax ginseng, a well-known herb in traditional medicine, have drawn attention. The active ingredients in Panax Ginseng, called ginsenosides, are thought to have adaptogenic qualities and are involved in the herb's mode of action. These substances might enhance general well-being by assisting the body in adjusting to stimuli. Furthermore, it is believed that panax ginseng affects the release of nitric oxide, a chemical that is essential for widening blood vessels and enhancing blood flow. Its reputation as a herb that encourages vigor and endurance may be attributed in part to this vascular function.

ADMINISTRATION & DOSAGE

Regarding dosage and method of administration, Panax Ginseng can be taken as teas, supplements, or as a component of energy beverages. It's important to remember that the right dosage can change depending on several variables, including age, health, and specific health objectives. To evaluate each person's tolerance, it is generally advised to begin with a smaller dose and raise it gradually.

GOAT HORN (EPIMEDIUM) WEED

Now let's turn our attention to Horny Goat Weed, or Epimedium as it is officially known. This plant has become well-known due to its possible health advantages, especially about erectile function. Icaridin, the active component of Horny Goat Weed, is thought to have a vasodilatory effect. This suggests that it might aid in blood vessel relaxation, resulting in an increase in blood flow to the vaginal region. Its traditional use as a natural treatment for sexual dysfunction stems from this method of action.

ADVANTAGES OF ERECTILE DYSFUNCTION

Horny Goat Weed supplementation may be of interest to men looking to improve erectile function because it can boost blood circulation in the pelvic region. It is crucial to stress that further research is required to completely understand the safety and efficacy of Horny Goat Weed for this purpose, even though some studies indicate a good influence. As with any herbal cure, it is best to speak with a medical practitioner before using it, particularly if you intend to use it as part of a treatment plan for a particular health issue.

Two herbal medicines that have drawn interest due to their possible health benefits are Panax ginseng and Horny Goat Weed. While Horny Goat Weed is explicitly linked to possible advantages for erectile function, Panax Ginseng is known for its adaptogenic qualities and influence on nitric oxide release.

CHAPTER FIVE

THOUGHTS AND ADVERSE REACTIONS

INCREASING BLOOD FLOW

Enhancing blood flow is essential to preserving general health and well-being. Enough blood flow guarantees that nutrients and oxygen reach all of the body's organs and tissues effectively. Engaging in frequent physical activity is a noteworthy way to improve blood flow. Exercises that encourage blood vessel dilatation, such as weight training and aerobic activities, lower the risk of cardiovascular problems and support healthy circulation. Additionally, by promoting vascular health, eating a balanced diet full of foods high in antioxidants and nutrients can help to enhance blood flow.

POSSIBLE RELATIONSHIPS

It is important to take into account the intricacy of the biochemical processes occurring in the human body while investigating possible interactions between various substances or treatments. Some chemicals can interact with one another and increase or decrease one another's effects. This is especially crucial when using prescription medications, herbal supplements, or other substances that support good health together. Before adding new components to a health routine, it is best to speak with a healthcare provider. They may offer tailored advice based on a person's unique medical problems and prescriptions.

TERRESTRIS TRIBULUS

The plant Tribulus Terrestris, which is frequently utilized in traditional medicine, has drawn interest due to its possible health advantages. Due to its frequent associations with testosterone-boosting qualities, it is a well-liked option for people looking to improve their athletic performance or take care of certain sexual health issues. Although some research indicates a favorable association between supplementing with Tribulus Terrestris and elevated testosterone levels, the results are not always definitive.

It is important to use herbal supplements with caution and to be aware of any potential adverse effects or interactions with other medications, just like you would with any other supplement.

PROPERTIES THAT BOOST TESTOSTERONE

Tribulus Terrestris is included in several dietary supplements due to its alleged ability to increase testosterone. It is significant to remember that different people react differently to these supplements, and that age, health, and pre-existing hormone levels can all have an impact on how well Tribulus Terrestris works. People should speak with a healthcare provider before starting Tribulus Terrestris to be sure it won't negatively impact their general health and to keep an eye out for any side effects.

USAGE INSTRUCTIONS

Following dosage recommendations is essential to maximizing the health advantages and lowering any potential hazards associated with supplements, especially those containing Tribulus Terrestris. Following the suggested dosage guidelines is essential because overindulging could have unfavorable consequences. To help the body adjust to the supplement, it's also a good idea to start with a smaller dose and raise it gradually as needed. It's crucial to keep an eye out for any indications of pain, allergic reactions, or drug interactions. Before introducing such supplements into their routines, people who are pregnant, nursing, or have pre-existing medical disorders should proceed with extra caution and seek advice from healthcare specialists. In conclusion, when thinking about using supplements like Tribulus Terrestris in one's health regimen, responsible and informed use is essential, along with professional advice.

CHAPTER SIX

RECIPES AND FORMULAS FOR HERBS

HERBAL TEAS FOR HEALTHY ERECTILE FUNCTION

For generations, people have used herbal teas as a natural way to support their overall health, including their erection. Many herbs are well known for their ability to improve circulation and promote reproductive health, two important aspects of treating erectile dysfunction. For example, ginseng is frequently added to herbal teas because of its adaptogenic qualities, which are thought to help the body adjust to stress and increase endurance.

Herbs like maca root and horny goat weed are also frequently used to mix because of their traditional medical history of treating problems with sexual function. These teas offer a comprehensive approach to promoting erectile health in addition to being tasty.

EXTRACTS AND TINCTURES

Herbal tinctures and extracts are concentrated versions of herbal medicines made by extracting the plant's active ingredients with alcohol or other solvents. These strong concoctions offer a practical and effective means of introducing herbal treatments into daily life. Herb extracts and tinctures such as tribulus terrestris and saw palmetto can be utilized for erectile dysfunction. Tribulus terrestris is thought to help boost testosterone levels, while saw palmetto may help keep the prostate healthy, which is crucial for general reproductive health. The ability to precisely control dosage using tinctures facilitates the customization of herbal therapies to meet specific needs.

BLENDS & SMOOTHIES USING HERBS

Blending herbs into smoothies is an inventive and delightful approach to take advantage of their possible health benefits. Herbal smoothies that combine elements that enhance hormonal balance, circulation, and general vigor can be customized to address specific issues connected to erectile health. Blend in fruits and other nutrient-dense ingredients, such as beetroot (high in nitrates that may improve blood flow) and maca root (said to have adaptogenic and libido-enhancing effects). This guarantees a varied intake of herbal compounds good for reproductive health in addition to giving the daily routine a delightful twist.

FORMULATING A CUSTOMIZED HERBAL REGIMEN

Creating a customized herbal regimen requires careful evaluation of each person's unique health requirements and preferences. This method acknowledges that every person's body reacts to herbs differently and that the efficacy of a customized protocol can be maximized. A vital first step is to consult with a licensed herbalist or healthcare provider. A detailed evaluation of the patient's lifestyle, general health, and any current medical issues is usually part of the process. Using this data, a customized concoction of herbal teas, tinctures, and smoothies can be created to target certain issues with erectile function. For best outcomes and to account for the evolving health state, routine monitoring and procedure modifications may be required. In the end, a customized herbal protocol encourages people to actively participate in their health, promoting a comprehensive strategy for wellness that goes beyond treating symptoms.

CHAPTER SEVEN

DIETARY GUIDELINES AND LIFESTYLE FACTORS

DIET'S IMPACT ON ERECTILE FUNCTION

Diet is essential for preserving general health and has an impact on many other areas of health, including erection health. To support optimal blood flow, hormone management, and cardiovascular health—all of which are factors that affect erectile function—a well-balanced and nutrient-rich diet is crucial. Fruits, vegetables, whole grains, and lean meats can all be found in diets high in these nutrients, which help the body's physiological functions associated with sexual health.

FOODS THAT HELP WITH IMPOTENCE

Some meals have been linked to improving sexual health in general and erectile function in particular. The vasodilator nitric oxide, which increases blood flow, is especially crucial for erectile function. Foods high in arginine, like legumes, seeds, and nuts, can increase the synthesis of nitric oxide. Furthermore, increased blood circulation has been connected to dark chocolate, which is high in flavonoids. Citrulline, found in fruits like watermelon, is converted by the body into arginine, which helps blood flow even more. Fish and flaxseeds include omega-3 fatty acids, which have anti-inflammatory qualities that may improve vascular health and, in turn, erectile performance.

FOODS TO STEER CLEAR OF

Dietary decisions can have a detrimental effect on erectile dysfunction. Diets heavy in cholesterol, trans fats, and saturated fats can impede blood flow, which is necessary for getting and keeping an erection, by narrowing blood vessels and causing atherosclerosis. Overindulgence in processed foods, sweetened beverages, and high-sodium meals can worsen cardiovascular problems and obesity, which can further impair erectile function.

Cutting back on these harmful foods is essential to preserving the health of your vascular system and promoting erectile function.

PHYSICAL ACTIVITY AND EXERCISE

A healthy lifestyle revolves around regular physical activity, which also positively affects erectile function. Exercise prevents erectile dysfunction by strengthening blood flow, improving cardiovascular health, and assisting in maintaining a healthy body weight. Cardiovascular fitness can be enhanced by resistance training as well as aerobic activities like swimming or running. Furthermore, exercise has been connected to the release of endorphins, which lessen stress and anxiety—two things that are frequently linked to problems in achieving sexual harmony.

TECHNIQUES FOR STRESS MANAGEMENT

Stress can cause hormonal imbalances and blood vessel constriction, which are major contributors to erectile dysfunction. It is imperative to include stress management strategies into one's lifestyle to maintain general health and, by extension, erectile function. Activities that assist in reducing stress and fostering calmness include gradual muscular relaxation, yoga, deep breathing techniques, and mindfulness meditation. Getting enough sleep is also essential for hormone balance and stress management. Creating a comprehensive strategy for stress management can have a favorable impact on one's physical and mental health, which will tangentially improve erectile function.

Sustaining the best possible erectile health depends critically on lifestyle choices including nutrition, exercise, and stress reduction. Well-being and sexual function can be enhanced by eating a nutritious, well-balanced diet, exercising frequently, and practicing good stress management. Making educated decisions on these areas of lifestyle might enable people to take charge of their erectile health and sustain fulfilling and healthy sexual relationships.

CHAPTER EIGHT

COMBINING CONVENTIONAL AND CONTEMPORARY METHODS

BLENDING TRADITIONAL MEDICAL PROCEDURES WITH HERBAL REMEDIES

To improve patients' overall well-being, healthcare providers must carefully combine conventional and modern treatments. A noteworthy feature of this integration is the combination of traditional medical treatments and natural therapies. The potential therapeutic effects of traditional herbal treatments, which have their roots in centuries-old practices, have gained acknowledgment. An approach to healthcare that is more comprehensive and individualized is made possible by incorporating these treatments into traditional treatment programs.

When it comes to chronic diseases, the benefits of using both herbal medicines and conventional treatments work well together.

For example, those with diabetes or hypertension may discover that taking herbal supplements in addition to their prescription drugs can improve their general health. To guarantee safety and efficacy, however, these integrations must be overseen by licensed healthcare specialists. When traditional and contemporary medicine works together, they can create a holistic treatment plan that takes care of a patient's symptoms as well as their underlying causes.

SPEAKING WITH MEDICAL EXPERTS

One of the most important components of successfully integrating old and modern approaches is consulting with healthcare specialists. When it comes to helping patients navigate the intricacies of integrating several modalities, healthcare providers are essential. Expert guidance on the suitability of herbal medicines in conjunction with prescription drugs, possible side effects, and the right dosage to prevent negative interactions can be obtained from them. This cooperative strategy promotes a patient-centered paradigm in which the knowledge of contemporary medical professionals and traditional healers is combined for the benefit of the patient's well-being.

TRACKING DEVELOPMENT AND MODIFYING APPROACHES

A continuing and dynamic aspect of integrated healthcare is tracking results and making necessary adjustments to strategies. Healthcare providers can decide whether changes are required based on regular evaluations of a patient's reaction to the integrated treatment plan. This flexibility is essential since different people react differently to integrated approaches. Continuous monitoring makes it possible to spot any unanticipated adverse effects or changes in health status, which makes it easier to intervene quickly to maximize the treatment plan's overall efficacy.

Preventive care is another area where traditional and modern methods are integrated, even beyond the therapeutic stage. Long-term well-being can be enhanced by encouraging patients to embrace lifestyle changes based on both conventional wisdom and modern health advice. To promote general health, this may entail a mix of dietary adjustments, exercise, and the use of herbal supplements. A more inclusive and thorough approach to healthcare that takes into consideration a variety of perspectives and practices is made possible by the cooperative efforts of healthcare professionals, traditional healers, and patients.

The fusion of conventional and modern methods in medicine is a beautiful synthesis of traditional knowledge and cutting-edge research. The cornerstones of this integrative paradigm include combining herbal therapies with conventional treatments, seeking advice from medical professionals, and regularly assessing results and modifying tactics. A more individualized and comprehensive approach to health and well-being can be provided to patients by healthcare professionals by embracing the benefits of both traditional and modern medicine.

CHAPTER NINE

CASE STUDIES AND TRIUMPHANT NARRATIVES

ACTUAL HERBAL MEDICINE EXPERIENCES

Many people from all around the world have offered inspiring first-hand accounts of their experiences using herbal treatments, demonstrating the effectiveness of these natural alternatives in fostering health and well-being. These experiences cover a broad spectrum of medical diseases, from simple illnesses like colds and stomach problems to more chronic conditions like arthritis and sleeplessness. A recurring motif in these narratives is the customized aspect of herbal medicines; people frequently recount how a particular herb or blend of herbs catered to their particular needs resulted in notable health advancements.

These stories demonstrate the variety of herbal therapies and the all-encompassing perspective they offer to healthcare.

Not only have people reported feeling better physically, but their general quality of life has also improved. These experiences highlight the value of including herbal medicines in addition to conventional medical treatments as part of an all-encompassing plan for health and wellness.

ACQUIRED KNOWLEDGE AND UNDERSTANDING

Using herbal treatments can lead to insightful and instructive discoveries and lessons. It's important to remember that consistency and patience are necessary. Herbal medicines frequently take time to enter the system and start working, in contrast to some conventional pharmaceuticals that could offer relief right away. To observe benefits, users usually stress how crucial it is to incorporate these remedies into daily routines and maintain a long-term commitment.

Furthermore, people frequently learn how important it is to comprehend their own bodies and distinct health profiles. They find the herbs that work best for their systems by making mistakes and trying different combinations. Through this process of self-discovery, people can establish a stronger bond with their health and become more proactive about their well-being.

RESOLVING FREQUENTLY ASKED QUESTIONS

Even with the increasing acceptance of herbal medicines, people still have common apprehensions and misgivings. The absence of established dosages and laws for herbal products is a common concern. Users often stress that to ensure the safe and suitable use of these medicines, it is crucial to consult with competent practitioners or herbalists. This cooperative approach guarantees a more knowledgeable and customized treatment plan while easing concerns about dosage unpredictability.

The possibility of interactions between conventional drugs and natural therapies is another prevalent issue.

To prevent any negative effects, users emphasize how crucial it is to have open contact with healthcare providers. The individual's well-being must be prioritized collaboratively and knowledgeably to bridge the gap between herbal and conventional therapy.

DISPELLING MYTHS REGARDING HERBAL TREATMENTS

The misconceptions that surround herbal treatments are sometimes the result of ignorance and false information. A common misconception is that using herbal medicines implies they don't have any scientific support. A great deal of research has been done on the pharmacological characteristics of many herbs, providing insight into their modes of action and their medical advantages.

There's also a misperception that there is a one-size-fits-all approach to using herbal treatments. Users emphasize how crucial it is to understand that herbal therapy is personalized and that what works for one person might not work as well for another. To maximize the benefits of herbal remedies, it is imperative to customize them to specific needs and situations.

Real-world experiences with herbal treatments offer a wealth of insights, insightful lessons, and success stories. Fostering a more knowledgeable and inclusive approach to healthcare that combines the benefits of both conventional and herbal treatment requires addressing prevalent issues and dispelling myths.